Medical School Multiple Mini Interview: Secrets for Success

James Wayne

Maximello Publishers
868, 141-6200 McKay Ave.
Burnaby, BC V5H 4M9
http://www.maximello.com

James Wayne
http://www.medicalschoolmmi.com

Printed in Canada

First Printing: August 2009

Cover design by David Wang

Wayne, James, 1984-
Medical school multiple mini interview : secrets for success / James Wayne.

Includes bibliographical references.
ISBN 978-0-9813492-0-6

1. Medical college applicants--Canada--Interviews--Study guides.
2. Medical colleges--Canada--Entrance examinations--Study guides.
I. Title.

R838.5.W39 2009 610.76 C2009-905458-2

TABLE OF CONTENTS

TABLE OF FIGURES

1. INTRODUCTION

Applying to medical school is an arduous, taxing, and frustrating process and the interview is a stressful situation in itself without the novel multiple mini interviews (MMI). The MMI is a recent innovation in medical school interviews that has caused dread, apprehension and fear in many medical school applicants. There are plenty of information on traditional interviews that range from the books on medical school and job interviews, and talking to doctors and medical students who have all been through the traditional interview. In contrast to traditional interviews, where information is replete, the MMI is very different and there are few resources. Information and experience are invaluable in making the medical school application process smoother and interview less stressful. This book aims to inform you about the MMI, help prepare you for the MMI, and to give you some tips and advice to get you ready for your MMI.

2. MMI BACKGROUND

Why is the traditional panel-style interview being replaced with the MMI?

The traditional panel-style interview can be influenced by the biases, expectations, and perspectives of the interviewers and do not necessarily predict the success of candidates upon completion of medical school (Harasymn et al. 1996, Eva et al. 2004b). A few years ago, studies started from McMaster University have provided evidence that the multiple mini interviews are better than the traditional panel-style interview in predicting the success of selected candidates for medical school (Eva et al. 2004a). The MMI has numerous strengths which led to several of Canada's medical schools to adopt it as a tool for selecting students. The MMI allows multiple testing of the candidate's ability and dilutes the effect of chance and interviewer bias. The MMI is standardized by structuring the MMI stations so that all the candidates respond to the same questions and the interviewers all receive common training and background information. The examiner can create virtually an infinite number of questions to test for personal attributes desired by the medical school. Candidates can recover from a poor performance on a particular station by moving to a new and independent interviewer. Scientific studies have found the MMI to be better at predicting pre-clerkship OSCE performance than traditional assessments (Eva et al. 2004b). In short, the MMI is a recent innovation in medical school interviews that is constantly evolving but has already been shown to be valid, reliable, and fairer in comparison to the traditional interview. The basic concept is to provide a standardized interview format in regards to the questions asked and method of evaluation.

What is the MMI (Multiple Mini Interview)?

The MMI is a recent innovation that has only existed for about five years with wider adoption in the last 2 years and is drastically different from the traditional interview. The MMI was developed in 2003 at McMaster University, used to select students in 2004 with the Northern Ontario Medical School, and in 2008 all five Western Canadian medical schools and five Eastern Canadian medical schools used the MMI.

The majority of Canadian medical schools now use the MMI. The University of British Columbia, University of Alberta, University of Calgary, University of Saskatchewan, University of Manitoba, Northern Ontario Medical School, Dalhousie University, Memorial University, McGill University, and McMaster Medical School all use the MMI. This is a recent phenomenon in which only two years ago, the opposite was true, only McMaster and the University of Calgary used the MMI and the rest of the Canadian medical schools continued to use the traditional interview. Australian medical schools are now also using the MMI.

The multiple mini interview (MMI) is a series of short interviews with a different interviewer each time. The purpose of the mini interviews is to assess personal traits or qualities desired by the medical school. In each mini interview, the candidate has two minutes to read a question/scenario and mentally prepare before entering the interview room. After entering the room the candidate is given eight minutes with an interviewer to answer the question. At the end of the interview, the interviewer uses the next two minute period to evaluate while the candidate moves to the next question. This process is repeated through 8 to 12 stations depending on the school. Some schools will also include rest stations. The total time for the interview is generally about 2 hours.

3. What to expect in an MMI?

Each medical school has variations in the implementation of the MMI, but they all follow a general procedure. The candidates arrive in a room (collecting room) where they will receive a name tag, separated into groups, and will be explained the process of the MMI. The name tag will have a number that will indicate the order and room in which you begin answering the MMI questions. On the name tag, the MMI group that you belong will also be written and the group is usually labeled by a color. Also on the name tag is your name and a photograph of you.

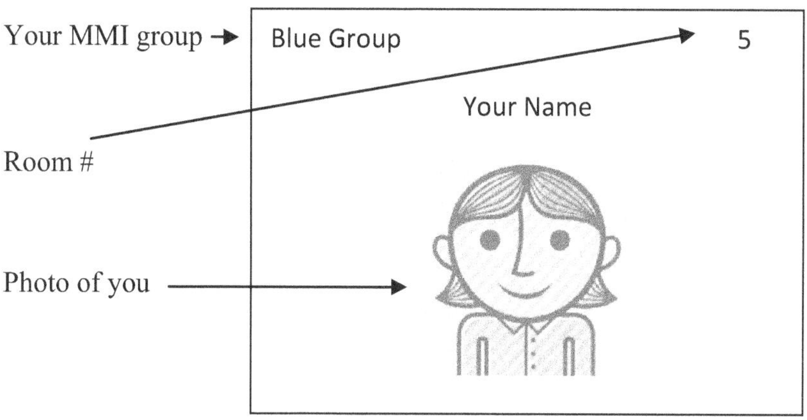

Figure 1 Diagram of MMI name tag

The applicants will line up according to the number assigned and written on the name tag. There will be about 8 to 10 questions so there will be about 8 to 10 applicants per group. The number of questions varies between the schools but most have 8 questions and some have 2 rest stations in addition to the questions where the applicant can rest.

The applicants will be taken from the collecting room to a long hallway with many rooms that are numbered.

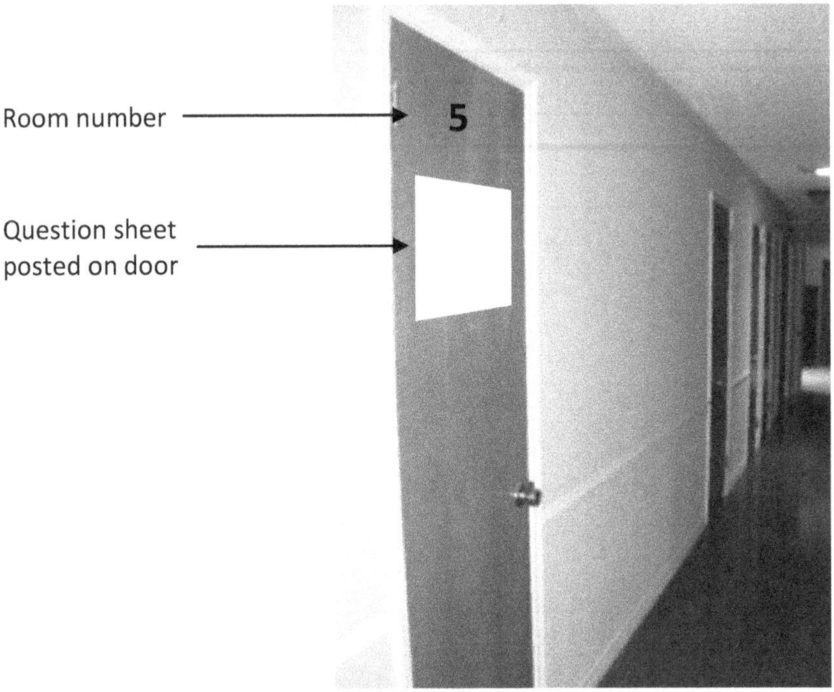

Figure 2 Typical MMI testing facility

Each room will have one interview question. The applicants stand in front of the room labeled with the same number that was assigned to them. A bell will ring and the applicant can read the question posted on the door of the room. The applicant will have two minutes to read and think about the question. A bell will ring at the end of the two minutes to signal the applicants to stop reading the question and to enter the room to answer the question.

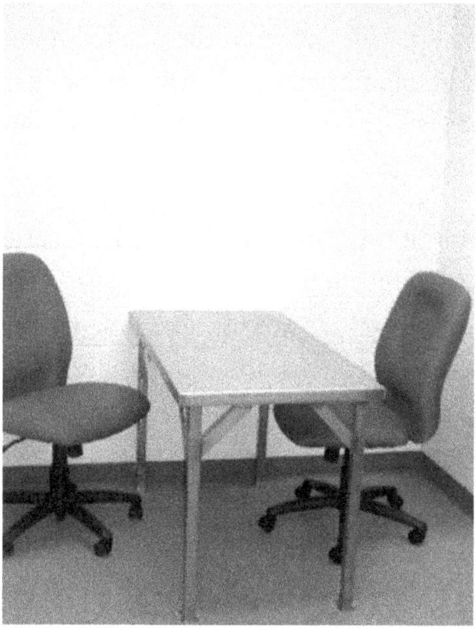

Figure 3 Typical multiple mini interview room

An interviewer will be inside the room. The applicant will have 8 to 10 minutes to answer the question depending on the medical school. A bell will ring to signal the time limit to answer the question and the applicant will leave the room. The interviewer will fill out the evaluation form for the applicant when the applicant has left the room. The applicant moves to the next door and begins reading the question for two minutes and the cycle is repeated until the applicant answers all the questions. As you progress through the questions, there may be one or more rest stations in which you can sit and rest for the time allotted for one interview question.

What are the MMI questions like?

MMI questions are usually a scenario that you can easily relate to and culminates with a specific question for you to answer. The scenarios are clearly written and unambiguous. The preamble is less than 100 words. There are no correct answers and there will be enough material for you to talk for eight minutes.

There will be prompting questions, which are a series of questions, usually three to five questions, designed to help you if you require it. The prompting questions are not provided to you but are given as a list to the interviewer. You can ask the interviewer for the prompting questions or the interviewer can offer them to you if they feel it would help you. Usually the interviewer will ask you the prompting questions after you finish your initial response. The prompting questions are provided one at a time and the interviewer is not allowed to deviate from the list of questions and so some of the questions may ask for things you have already mentioned in your initial answer.

The feeling while you wait for the bell to ring and begin the MMI

You will arrive at the medical school and walk along the entrance and down a hallway while following the signs to the registration booth. At the registration booth you provide the documents the school has sent and requested you to complete for submission on the day of the interview. In exchange for the documents you will receive a name tag to hang around your neck and it might even have a photo of you that you submitted earlier by e-mail and a page full of small stickers that have your name and a number printed on each sticker. You are told to sit in a common area with rows of seats filled by other applicants dressed in dark suits who are also wearing name tags, holding stickers and waiting. There is a table full of water bottles that you will walk by to pick up a bottle for yourself before finding a seat. If you're lucky, there will be some current medical students available to chat with you to reassure you to not be nervous and to answer any questions you might have about the medical school and program. The medical student disclaims that nothing you discuss with him or her will affect your admission. You will probably chat with a few fellow applicants and medical students. You have about ten or twenty minutes before the MMI orientation begins and you're allowed to use the washroom to freshen up, relieve any nervous energy, and to go the washroom so you won't need to during the interview. You look at your sheet of stickers and wonder what it is used for. The time for the interview orientation approaches and you are split into a group of about ten people, given a number and color that you realized is printed on your stickers and name tag, and line up in a predetermined number sequence. The orientation leader explains the instructions of the MMI and the purpose of the stickers.

Instructions for the MMI:

The interview orientation leader will verbally describe the instructions and if you're fortunate they may even have a PowerPoint presentation as part of the explanation.

There will be eight applicants and a leader who will meet in the collecting room where you wait and receive instructions. Then you will be taken to the interview rooms and you stand in front of the door that you have been assigned. A bell will ring and you will have 2 minutes to read the question before another bell will ring to signal the end of the 2 minutes and you can enter the room to begin your interview with the interviewer. You will have 8 minutes in the interview room with the interviewer. When you are seven minutes into the station, you will hear a bell to let you know that you have a minute left to finish answering the question. Then another bell will ring when you have spent 8 minutes in the room and this will signal the end of the station. You will then proceed to the next room and have another 2 minutes to read the question. This will continue until all the stations are complete. Then you will return to the room in which we had the orientation for a short debriefing.

The stickers are to be given to the interviewer at each station who will place the sticker on your evaluation sheet. It is important that you remember to give the sticker to each interviewer, the orientation leader reminds everyone. The orientation leader suggests that everyone bend open the corners for each of the stickers to make it easier for you to remove the sticker for the interviewer because every candidate will invariably be nervous and fumbles with the sticker as he or she tries to give the sticker to the interviewer. After the explanation of the MMI procedure all the applicants wait in the lineup for the group leaders to bring the applicants to the interview rooms. The applicants are taken to a narrow hallway full of doors with pages stuck on the doors and seats in front of each door. The applicants are lead down the hallway of doors and stand in front of the door with the number that corresponds with the number on their name tag. The applicants are told to stand with their backs to the door and not to read the sheet of paper that was stuck on the door. The applicants stare across the hallway, look and smile at other applicants who are staring back and waiting. You notice a few nervous applicants taking deep breaths and crossing their hearts. You wait for the bell to ring to start the first question out of the series of multiple mini interview questions. The bell finally rings and you turn around to read the question. You read the question and ponder about the question and think about what to say to the interviewer. You look around and all the applicants are staring intently at the door and reading the question. Some applicants are dancing around while they're thinking and oblivious to everyone and everything else while others are frantically writing notes. You finished reading the question with plenty of time to spare and have thought of almost everything you could think of and the bell rings and you open the door to enter a small room with white walls, no windows, and a small table in the middle and a chair on either side.

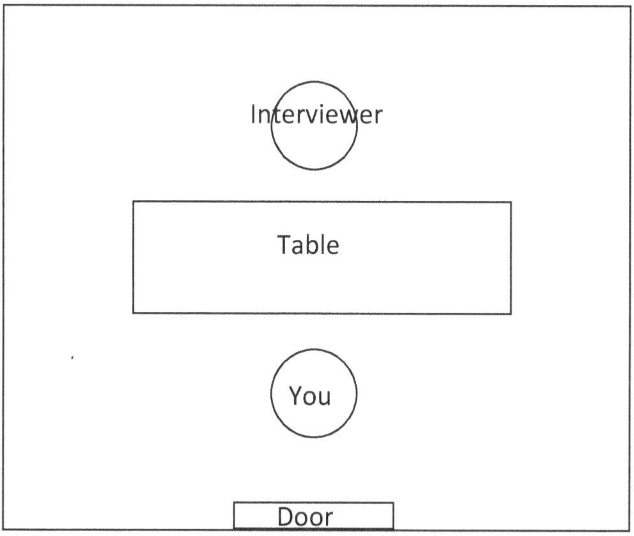

Figure 4 Layout of MMI Room

The interviewer is sitting in the far chair behind the table and gets up as you say hello and you walk towards her to shake her hand. She invites you to sit down and asks for your sticker. You fumble to find the sticker and peel just one sticker to the interviewer who takes the sticker and places it on a blank evaluation sheet. You wait for the interviewer to start the interview and she smiles and looks back and asks if you had a chance to read the question and points to a sheet of paper on the desk that is a photocopy of the question sheet that was on the door. You reply that you have had a chance to look at the question and she invites you to start whenever you're ready. You talk about everything you thought of outside of the room and you managed to fill a few minutes. But there are several more minutes left and the interviewer asks a question and you are inspired to talk some more until you have finished expressing your thoughts. The interviewer again asks another question and you talk again. Now that you're done talking the interviewer asks if you have anything else you would like to add and invites you to look at the question sheet again if you want. You look at the question sheet again but can't think of anything else to add. She tells you that is okay and that we'll just wait for the bell to signal the end of the station. You remember you were told in the interview orientation that you're not allowed to talk to the interviewer about anything other than the question and that the interviewer will not respond to any attempts at chit chatting even if there is an awkward silence. The interviewer smiles at you as you stare back at her while you wait for the station to end. There is a pitcher of ice water and a stack of plastic cups. You pour yourself a cup of water and didn't' realize how thirsty you really felt until the soothing cold water coats your tongue. You look around the room as a distraction to the awkward silence. Suddenly the buzzer rings to signal the end of the station and you feel a sense of relief as you pop out of the chair to shake the interviewer's hand and thank her while you rush out of the room and close the door to see the applicant in the next door come out and rush to the next room. You rush to the next room to maximize the time to read and think about the next question because you know the buzzer that signaled the end of the question also signaled the beginning of the two minutes to read the next question. You continue this sequence again for another three stations and you begin to feel tired but the nervous and anxious energy begins to subside as you get into the swing of things and feel like you know how the MMI works. If you're lucky, the university has a rest station at about the half way point and you get to sit and relax for eight minutes, use the washroom and maybe even chat with a medical student. Then you continue again through another four stations. As you near the end of the stations you begin to count and look forward to the last station. You feel tired and want to get the stations over with as you near the second to last station. When you finish all the stations you feel a sense of relief followed immediately by a feeling of surprise that it is all over and it wasn't as bad or as long as you thought it would be. As you move out of the interview area you start to feel really tired mentally and physically. You start to think that the MMI lasted for a long time but when you do the math you realize it lasted only for an hour and a half. You overhear some other applicants talking out loud about feeling tired from the interview and feel a sense of relief that it wasn't only you who felt this way. As you enter the resting room to fill out evaluation forms a lady walks around with a plate of cookies and you gladly take a cookie to fuel yourself with sugar and to treat yourself for finishing the multiple mini interview. The interviews are done and you are free to go or to continue to attend the activities and tours planned by the school.

4. Marking Scheme

The MMI's are marked on a scale of 1 to 10, 1 to 4 or another combination depending on the school. The interviewers are encouraged to use as much of the scale as possible to create clear distinctions between applicants. In general, the interviewers are considering the strength of the arguments and answers, ability to communicate clearly, concisely, and in an organized manner, the applicant's suitability as a physician, and the overall impression of the applicant and his or her response.

McMaster's medical school marking scheme can be found on their website (http://fhs.mcmaster.ca/mdprog/interviews.html). Each interview question is marked on three criteria. The interviewer is to rank the applicant on each of the criteria as being in the top or bottom percentile. In McMaster University, the applicants have been ranked in the top 1%, 3%, 5%, 10%, 15%, 25%, 35%, 50%, or 75 % of applicants or in the bottom 25% of applicants. The three criteria are:

1. Score of the communication skills the applicant displayed during the station
2. Score of the strength of the applicant's arguments presented during the station
3. Rating of the applicant's suitability for a career in medicine based on the brief encounter during the station

   There is also a score for the applicant's overall performance on the station and room for comments

The important thing to note is that the evaluation sheets are in general looking at a few common broad categories and the applicants are ranked on a scale of relative performance.

Please note that an applicant scoring unsatisfactory in one checklist item does not mean the applicant has failed. An applicant doing poorly in one section can be compensated for by doing well in other sections.

Some of the attributes that may be considered during the evaluation center around qualities desired in a health care professional. A good description and definition of some of the attributes desired for a health care professional can be found on the University of Sydney website (http://www.medfac.usyd.edu.au/futurestudent/applicant/mmi_interviewertrain_09.pdf). Some of the attributes include integrity, respect for diversity, sensitivity to the needs of others and establish rapport, self control, tact and diplomacy, conscientiousness, effective communicator, demonstrates insight, effective decision maker, information manager, ability to make a shared plan, self directed learner, and understanding the role of health professionals in society.

About the Interviewers

The interviewers are generally trained by the medical school about a week prior to the interview. In general, the training provides background and evaluation information on the medical school, admission and interview and includes a brief overview of the current curricula, overview of the admission procedures to the medical school program, practical aspects of being an interviewer in the MMI, and applying the scoring system. Each interviewer will only evaluate one question and will repeatedly evaluate many applicants and their responses to the single question they were assigned. The initial few applicants of the interview period will set the expectation for the interviewers. The interviewers are generally medical students, faculty, and community members and you will not know the background of the interviewers. The interviews will introduce themselves by their name, so for example, John Smith instead of Dr. Smith or Professor Smith.

Prompting Questions

The use of the prompting question may affect your evaluation. Prompting questions help the applicant to cover the different points of the question and allow the applicant a fair opportunity to show the applicant's thinking. If the applicant does not use the prompting questions as a crutch to get them to answer the question then the applicant should not be penalized. In general, the applicant should try their best to answer the question and use the prompting questions when necessary.

Useful Training Exercise

It is a useful exercise to find a few friends or family members to answer an MMI question and for you to evaluate them. You should video record the interview, preferable at an angle to view both the interviewer and the responder. By going through the evaluation on someone else, you will gain insight on the thought process of the interviewer and this will give you a better understanding of factors interviewers will be evaluating. When you view the video of the interview, you will notice your own facial reactions as an interviewer in response the answers of the other person and you can objectively learn from the strength and weaknesses of the responder's body posture/language, delivery, and answer.

5. Nuances in MMI Between Schools

Although the MMI is similar in concept, the implementation varies between the schools, and there are nuances that make every MMI different between the schools. In order to give you an idea of the differences in implementation of the MMI, we will go through a couple of schools. In general, the differences increase the further the schools are apart in the east and west direction. Schools on the west side of Canada tend to have interviewers that don't show emotions, responses or won't engage in small talk during the interview while the opposite is true as you move east across Canada where the interviews may have similar questions but the interviewers are more willing to show emotions, respond to the applicant's response and engage in small talk. The differences are highlighted by comparing the University of Calgary in Alberta to the University of British Columbia in British Columbia. There are many nuances even though these schools are in the two most western and neighboring Canadian provinces and would be expected to be most similar in MMI implementation.

University of Calgary

In the University of Calgary, the verbal MMI consists of 9 stations. At each station, you are given 2 minutes to read the scenario, then 8 minutes with the interviewer. U of C allows note taking with a pencil and paper provided before each question. The University of Calgary also has an additional written MMI station where you write two essays based on essay questions, statistics, articles, and pictures provided in a booklet. The essays are done on computer. The University of Calgary is the only school in Canada that has a written MMI station. A written MMI station has generally been held at the Library Commons in the Health Science Centre. There are 2 questions and you are given 60 minutes to complete your written answers. You are responsible for managing your time appropriately. Food or drinks are not allowed in the computer area. Earplugs are recommended if you tend to be distracted by noise, especially from the typing of other candidates. You can follow the link to thc Univcrsity of Calgary that provides more information on their MMI (http://medicine.ucalgary.ca/undergrad/ume/mmi).

University of British Columbia

The University of British Columbia has a more direct approach to the MMI and any presentations or social events are at a separate time and venue from the MMI. There are no pencils or papers allowed to jot down your thoughts for each question, so all your mental preparation has to be done in your head.

More information about the MMI at the University of British Columbia can be found by viewing the following link:
http://www.med.ubc.ca/education/md_ugrad/MD_Undergraduate_Admissions/MD_Undergraduate_Interviews.htm

Pictures illustrating the implementation of an MMI at the University of British Columbia are available on the University of British Columbia website at the following link:

http://www.med.ubc.ca/education/md_ugrad/MD_Undergraduate_Admissions/MD_Undergraduate_Interviews/Interview_Process_Demonstration.htm

6. APPROACH TO ANSWERING MMI QUESTIONS

A way to approach the MMI is to not use any pencils or papers to jot down your thoughts for each question, so all your mental preparation will be done in your head. The two minutes prior to answering the question as a chance to read the question, calm down, and brainstorm some ideas that come to mind when you read the question. Then go in, with some ideas that you've thought of and let them flow forward. Another approach is to use pencil and paper to jot down ideas and remember certain ideas, try to organize it, and try to go through everything in the interview. The drawback of the second approach is the tendency to be not as organized as you would have liked it to be because of the time constraints. Also the thoughts are not as complete as something that flows freely from the mind, and there is a pressure of trying to produce everything that was pre-thought out so it produces a less natural and more stagnant response. The style of letting your thoughts flow tends to be more natural, engaging, persuasive and can change with the reaction of the interviewer and the follow up questions. These other elements are important in the MMI because the interviewers are also measuring the softer skills of communication and add to the overall impression of the candidate. Hence, it is important to be relaxed and natural, while communicating persuasively, logically, and in an organized manner.

What to do in the two minutes before answering the question?

During the two minutes provided to read the question, the amount of time spent reading the question will be very short. The rest of the time in the two minute period should be used to think and brainstorm ideas that come to mind when you read the question. At the same time that you're thinking, you should be taking deep breaths to calm yourself and keep yourself relaxed. If you have the jitters and want to move to relax, now is the time to move around on the spot to help you relax and think. You might want to move your feet or perform other movements to make you feel in your zone while you're thinking. You don't need to worry about other people seeing you because everyone else will be doing their own thing and being focused on answering their own question. You might even inspire other people to relax and be themselves while they're thinking about their own question.

When you're running low on ideas, it is a good idea to read the question again to see if it will inspire more ideas and to make sure that you are really answering the question that is being asked. Sometimes there are questions that are aimed to test if you've actually read and answered the question being asked. When you've exhausted your ideas and you feel your time is running low, you should try to summarize the entire passage into one sentence framed as the question being asked. Think of that one question summary of the station when you walk into the room. While you're in the room answering the question, occasionally recall the question to check if you are answering the question and use it as a goal to stimulate further thoughts. Framing the question into one sentence focuses you when you answer the question and makes sure you won't forget the question or go off track. You are able to read the question while you're in the room, but you don't want be wasting time or be caught off guard in that situation.

You should wear a watch when you do the interview and check periodically to make sure you have enough time or to gauge the amount of time you spend answering and preparing for questions. You should check your watch at the beginning of the two minutes so you know how much time you have left to think and prepare for the question. The moment you are about to open the door to the room, you should have a look at your watch to get an idea of the start time so you can take a glance at your watch during the interview station to see the amount of time left to answer the question. It is okay to have a minute remaining before the buzzer signals the end of the question. The minute will go by very fast and it won't seem like a long wait before the buzzer signals you to leave the room. The minute wait will be just enough time to rest after your question and to let the answer sink in with the interviewer. A check on the watch will confirm that you are on track in terms of time. You don't want to end much too early as you'll have a very long silent period and you may give the impression of an incomplete answer. The questions generally are designed to give you enough to talk about to fill up the allotted time. The follow up questions will generally give enough momentum to help you make the time allotted for the question. During the silent period of waiting for the buzzer, getting a glass of water to drink is a good distraction to fill the awkward silence and it will give you a chance to calm down and to wet your tongue. Drink moderately but not too much because you won't have time to go to the washroom until you reach a break station if it is available.

Posture and Body Position in the MMI Room

While you're in the room answering questions, you should keep both feet flat on the ground, your hands neatly on your lap and sit leaning slightly forward. When you keep both your feet flat on the ground it helps to maintain composure and feel calm. This is a neutral position. Other positions such as crossing your legs will create a large physical gap between you and the interviewer which could hamper rapport and may be culturally insensitive because some cultures believe that a person crossing their legs is a sign of lack of respect for the interviewer. Moreover, keeping the same body position in each interview question builds a routine, removes a factor in your thinking and ensures that you are in the correct body position each time. Placing your hands on your lap prevents your body from performing unnecessary hand gestures that may be distracting to the interviewer and detract from your message. Often times the interview room is very small and excessive hand gestures may intrude on the interviewer's personal space while you think you are simply emphasizing or illustrating a point. When a very important and natural hand gesture occurs, you can let your hands move but after you've made your point, place your hands back on your lap. This habit will filter out unnecessary hand gestures and only let the important hand gestures be expressed which will make your message much more clear and powerful. When you sit and lean slightly forward it gives a more attentive and positive impression to the interviewer and it helps to keep your posture.

You should have a good posture while you are sitting and when you're standing because you will give a better impression, look and feel more confident. Good posture should be practiced at home to develop into a habit so you will not be distracted by consciously reminding yourself to have proper posture and can put all your effort into answering the MMI questions on the day of the interview. Methods to practice and improve posture at home prior to the interview are discussed in the training preparations at home section.

Eye contact with the interviewer is very important because you want to engage the interviewer and eye contact is one of the most important factors in getting and keeping your interviewer's attention. Since you will most likely be in a small room you don't want to stare at the interviewer or harbor hostility in your eye contact because it will be magnified in part due to the close proximity and direct seating arrangement. Smiling is also very important, especially when you first enter the room and greet the interviewer. Under the stress of the environment, many people forget to smile and may even have a serious or hostile expression, which can lower the score for the applicant because the interviewer is partly looking for social skills and making the other person feel comfortable while communicating.

Tips that'll be useful during the MMI

Different schools have different etiquette in regards to knocking on the door before you enter the room. Some have a habit of knocking while others don't really care. The moment you enter the room, you make eye contact, greet the interviewer, give a firm handshake, remember to give the interviewer your sticker, and then sit down. Many applicants fumble when removing the stickers or forget to give the sticker to the interviewers, and the interviewers often forget to remind the applicant. A tip to avoid forgetting or fumbling to remove the sticker is to loosen the edges of the stickers prior to the interview when you are waiting in the waiting room. Preparing the stickers will also occupy you when you're in the waiting room and help to calm you down. You can fold the sticker sheet and place it in your pocket to avoid the nervous gestures created by the temptation to play with the sticker sheet while holding on to it.

When leaving the station, you should give eye contact, shake the interviewer's hand, say thank you, and leave the room. You don't need to dawdle because the interviewer is expecting you to leave and you'll be wasting your time that should be using to read the next question.

Do not try to repeat or become circular when you run out of things to say as it will only make your message less clear, make you look less competent and confident, bore and lose the attention of the interviewer. It is better to state your points and have silence while you think of your next point then to repeat your points in the hopes of finding something else to say. You can ask the interviewer for follow up questions if you are struggling to find new material to talk about.

7. Types of MMI Questions

The span of questions for the MMI can be immense and even infinite but there are always a few categories of MMI questions that students can prepare for in terms of material and framework for answering certain types of questions.

The main types of MMI questions include, ethical – scenario based questions, society or current events questions, spontaneous – creative questions, getting to know you personally questions, and do you know the school questions. The delivery of the question can take on a few forms and include, direct questions, interactive chatting, interrogator and evaluator in the same room, and role playing questions.

Ethical-scenario based questions

Most of the questions are ethical based and are asked in a scenario in which you need to respond, form an opinion or most importantly to discuss both sides and weigh both sides of the problem. It is more important to discuss the reasons, the factors involved, views of both sides, and to come to the best conclusion possible based on the reasons and factors considered even though it may not be perfect because they will have questions that are very contentious, controversial and many competing factors and there won't be an easy answer. They will add competing factors to make sure that the problem is complicated enough that you won't have a simple answer. The interviewer may add pressure and press for a solid decision or action. An example could be a situation where a father requests the physician for an invasive procedure for his teenage daughter but the daughter refuses the test. The applicant is asked if he or she would provide the test. The situation is confounded by the independence of the daughter, right of the parent over the child, ability for the child to understand the procedure and consequences, invasiveness of the test, cost to society, fairness of allocation of resources, and the opinion of the mother. Outlining the issues is a significant aspect of answering such a question and the conflicting issues can be difficult to resolve. Possible options in this situation can include finding the opinion of the mother, seeking a legal consultation of the rights of the parent and the child, facilitation of the negotiation between the father and daughter, and providing time for them to resolve the issues and for the father to stabilize emotionally.

In general the first task in an ethical-scenario type of question is to find the issues being asked in the question and to address the issues. A good framework for ethical-scenario type of questions is to consider the right of independence or autonomy of the individual, the benefit to the individual, any harm to others, and equality or fairness to society or others. A strong support for answering ethical questions is to always consult with the legal system because the law often encompasses some solutions to ethical problems; a physician cannot disobey the law and must work in the boundaries of the law. To better understand the ethical considerations and legal advice, there are a number of resources available that will analyze many common clinical ethical cases and are used by health care professionals in learning to deal with ethical problems. The first is a book written by a clinician and expert in ethics and is called "Doing Right: A Practical Guide to Ethics for Medical Trainees and Physicians" by Philip C. Hebert. This book provides a framework to deal with clinical ethical problems and illustrates the analysis of these ethical problems with actual case reports. Another useful resource is a series of articles written by the Canadian Medical Association (www.cma.ca) under the section of policies and guidelines that discusses many common clinical ethical problems by providing a background of the problem, opinions of the issues, legal perspective of the problem and suggestions on dealing with the problem. By reading these resources you will develop a mindset in approaching ethical issues, and have an idea of where the law stands on the issue and based on the suggestions you will learn to think like a health care professional in dealing with the issues.

Society or current events questions

There may be questions that are based on events that are important to the city and in the news a lot. You need to be regularly reading the newspaper or watching the news to keep up to date on issues that are important in the city, country and world so that you will be prepared to comment on them or at least have a level of awareness of the issue in case they ask you. Reading news articles will provide a background and awareness of the issues. It is useful to regularly read the opinion articles in the newspaper and the letters to the editors to view different people's opinion on the topic to expand and to understand the arguments and perspectives on issues.

There are often questions on the health care system, areas of strength, areas for improvement and understanding of the Canadian health care system and comparing it to other health care systems in the world. You will need to understand the Canadian health care system and obtaining background information can be done through the Health Canada website where there are pdf documents describing the Canadian health care system. You will want to learn about the strengths, problems of the Canadian health care system and ideas proposed to improve the Canadian health care system. This can be done by searching websites, reading books, and being aware of news articles in the newspaper or magazines such as the Economists which often provides a good description of the problem and proposed solutions. For example, a major strength of the Canadian health care system is that universal health care is available to all citizens and is free at the point of use but this leads to the problem of long wait lists and possibly untimely access to health care services. One proposed solution is based on the observations that waitlists are longer for some specialists than others and by moving patients from doctors with long waitlists to doctors with shorter waitlists, the waitlist times can be made to be more reasonable. In other words, a more efficient allocation of resources would resolve some of the problems. Another issue with the health care system is the escalating cost of drugs which is one of the fastest growing and most significant health care expenditure for the country. A possible solution may be for the country to purchase pharmaceuticals in bulk to gain bargaining power to negotiate lower costs and work with pharmaceutical companies. An unlikely but useful area to obtain a quick overview of the problems and solutions on health care systems are from videos on YouTube. There are many videos on YouTube that provides information on health care systems, problems and solutions, health care systems of different countries, expert and people's opinions on the issue. The videos are often short, often entertaining, and compresses a lot of important information in a multimedia format.

Spontaneous – creative questions

There will be creative questions that test your critical thinking and will sometimes appear as if the exam question creator wanted to make a question that the interviewee will never think of and have them think on the spot. Usually, the questions are fun and you can think of ideas on the spot. You must relax and let your ideas flow and grasp and expand on ideas that first come to your mind. An example of such a question would be choosing a set of given items to survive if you are marooned on an island. There will be times in which the question will be scenario based and revolves around working with other people and enquires about your approach to resolving a problem. Creative scenarios are often fun but may surprise inexperienced applicants. The thought process and logic of the answer is primarily being evaluated by the interviewer. Your values and priorities that guide your decisions will be noted. The way you function in a team may be evaluated depending on what is provided by your answer.

Getting to know you personally questions

There will be questions that are very open ended and are aimed at knowing more about you as a person. An example question may be, to ask you to describing your perfect day and explain the things that make it special for you. There is no right or wrong answer and the interviewer is simply trying to understand you better. These types of questions are generally very relaxed and the interviewer is interested in listening to you share your interests, hobbies, and experiences.

Do you know the school questions

Sometimes the schools have a new program or new method of teaching or a vision that is unique to the school. The schools may ask questions to see if you are aware of the unique feature or aspect that is important to the school. For example, if the school has a campus or program in rural areas or wants to train more rural physicians, they may ask questions to probe your understanding of the rural program, understanding of small towns, and even ask you to weigh the strength and weaknesses of such a program, or the effectiveness of the program. If rural medicine is an important theme in the school, they may even ask for suggestions on providing patient care to rural areas.

Delivery of the questions

Direct Question

Most the questions are delivered by providing a preamble and asking a direct question. Sometimes the question is very simple or is even a yes or no question despite a long preamble. In general, the interviewer will expand and ask deeper questions after you respond with your initial impressions of the question and preamble.

Interrogator and evaluator in the same room

Most questions are asked with a single interviewer and evaluated by the same interviewer. However, there are questions in which there are two interviewers in the same room. You will be introduced to the two interviewers but one will sit in front of you and ask questions while the other interviewer will be in the back observing and evaluating and won't say much but will be writing a lot in a notepad. The interviewer who is not taking notes will be better able to react and respond to your answers and may even ask questions based on your response while the other person observes, takes notes, and evaluates. In general, you will only need to pay attention and maintain eye contact with the interviewer asking the question and you will only need to deal with the other interviewer when you enter and leave the room. The other interviewer will usually be too busy taking notes and evaluating and won't be providing much eye contact anyways.

Role Playing Questions

When you read the question on the piece of paper in front of the door, the preamble will look like a scenario based question except there will be a note saying the question is a role playing question and the last sentence will say something to the effect that there will be a person in the room playing the role mentioned in the preamble and you are to respond and interact with this actor or actress. When you enter the room, you will generally meet an interviewer who is an evaluator and will take notes in the background while you interact with the actor/actress. The actor/actress will be in the room and you will speak with the actor/actress. The degree of acting varies. There may be no props or any acting or any special make up or costume. The actor/actress may simply be in plain clothes and may not necessarily resemble the character you imagine him or her to be from reading the question. The person level of response from the actor/actress is variable. On the other hand, some role playing questions may be on the other end of the spectrum of hiring professional actors and actresses and using props and make up. Due to the range of possibilities, you should be prepared and not be surprised to encounter a role playing question ranging from minimal acting to a dramatic acting scene.

Summary of Types of Questions

The types of the questions covered by the MMI are:

- ethical – scenario based questions
- society or current events questions
- spontaneous – creative questions
- getting to know you personally questions
- do you know the school questions

The questions can be delivered the following forms:

- direct question
- interrogator and evaluator in the same room
- role play questions

8. PREPARATION PRIOR TO INTERVIEW

Preparation for the MMI is very important in order to do well and feel confident. The earlier you prepare the better you will feel and perform on the interview. Preparations should start at least three months before the interview. There are also certain considerations and things you should do the last few days and on the day of the interview to ensure that you are in your peak performance for interview day.

Three months before the interview

The MMI is a type of interview that you can practice and prepare for but will require more time to prepare because it involves practicing and getting into the mindset of answering MMI type of questions. There are materials that you can read to give you ideas and substance to talk about during the MMI. The earlier you read the material the more time you will have to digest and to allow your mind to subconsciously blend it into being a part of you so that you can easily, casually and confidently bring up and use the information during the interview. In addition, allotting more time will allow you to read more material and hopefully you will retain more information so that you may be able to recall enough information to answer in the multiple mini interview.

Mock MMI Practice

The first mock MMI you try is to get an idea of the type of questions, the experience of responding for eight minutes in a small room, reading and preparing a response to a question in two minutes, and the stress and stamina required to answer many questions in rapid succession. The first mock MMI should be video recorded and will serve as a baseline or your starting point before preparation. The second mock MMI should be performed after you've prepared for the MMI and should be video recorded. After the second mock MMI, you will review the recordings to find and write down on a notepad all the strengths and things you did well and the weaknesses and areas of improvements. Try to work on these areas of improvements and continue doing the things that were your strengths.

Mock MMI Simulation Conditions

Mock MMI exams are important to your preparation and should be done under MMI conditions as much as possible. The mock MMI should be performed in a room that most mimics the actual MMI room. So you should find a small room, preferably with white walls and with few furnishings except for a small table and two chairs on either side of the table. Try to post the questions with one question per page on the door to the room. In the real MMI, each question is printed on a separate piece of paper. The practice MMI in this book is designed have the same appearance as the real MMI. In the real MMI, the question sheets are taped on the door, but in a practice setting this is not necessary and inconvenient. The solution is provided in the practice MMI at the end of this book. Simply read the question printed in the book outside the room during the two minute period. Go inside the room and give the book to the mock interviewer so he or she can flip the page and read you the prompting questions when you need them. After you finish answering the questions and the time limit is up, you can take the book back out the room and read the next question. Before you begin the practice MMI, the mock interviewer can cut the interviewer evaluation sheet at the end of the book to give you a score for each question. The mock interviewer would be filling out the evaluation sheet while you read the next question outside the room.

Training and Preparation at Home

The bulk of the training for the multiple mini interviews can be done at home as you practice, review material, and generate positive habits that will carry through on the day of the interview so you don't need to pay attention to certain behaviors when you are stressed at the interview. Videotaping your practice interviews can be an invaluable tool to receive objective and private feedback and to monitor your progress. Videotaped interviews are an excellent tool to detect and help rectify distracting mannerisms and to check on posture. Proper posture will help in providing a positive and confident first impression. Proper breathing is important to produce better articulation. Proper posture and breathing is something that needs to be trained over time in order to be subconscious and a natural part of you on interview day.

Videotape Interview Practice

When you videotape yourself during practices, pay attention to filler words such as "uh", "um", "like", "so yeah", and "you know" and try to minimize your use of such words as it detracts from professionalism which is something the interviewers are looking for in their evaluation. In addition, it detracts from communication of your ideas which is another factor that the interviewers are evaluating. A method to give you an idea of the degree of the problem is to count the number of filler words in your video and work to minimize the tally of filler words with each practice. Mannerisms and unnecessary gestures should also be removed from your interviewing habits. A tip to pick up such mannerisms is to fast forward your videotape of your practice interview and these mannerisms will become very apparent. These mannerisms are very hard to correct because they are a part of your habit and you will most likely not be thinking of such things under the stress of the interview or thinking about such things will hamper your interview performance. So you should start early to give yourself lots of time for your preparations, to find these mannerisms through videotaped practices, and to work on these mannerisms over time.

Posture

A good posture for sitting and standing will give a better impression. Good posture can be practiced at home so that on interview day you can focus on the question and not add unnecessary stress. Practicing and training your body at home will generate a habit that will carry through to the interview. Doing posture exercises will also make you feel better and confident and has the added benefit of being a method to reduce stress accumulated in your daily life. A common exercise used for posture and relaxation in yoga and by actors/actresses is the rag doll exercise.

Posture Exercise

The rag doll exercise will clear your mind, relax your body, and help you find a comfortable, straight-up posture. The rag doll exercise is done by first standing straight in a relaxed, upright position. Stand up tall and inhale as your raise your hands straight into the air above your head. Relax, exhale and lower your hands to your feet while keeping your legs straight. Be sure to release your neck so that it feels loose. While you are bent over, gently sway back and forth. Don't forget to breathe. Let your body hang in this position while you breathe deeply and slowly for at least five breaths. When you have relaxed into this position, gently begin to roll up from the back of your knees, through your buttocks, and all the way through your spine, one vertebra at a time. Continue to slowly raise your body one vertebra at a time and only raise your head when you have raised your shoulders. Once you are upright, be sure to take a deep breath and relax your shoulders on the exhale. The process of raising your body up should take at least 10 seconds. The position at the end of the rag doll exercises is the body's natural upright posture. Performing this exercise at least once a day on a daily basis will improve your posture.

Breathing

Breathing is essential to life and we breathe from the moment of birth to the time we die. Unfortunately, when we get anxious we often forget to breathe properly. Learning to control and use your breathing constructively can be an enormous aid in times of stress. Breathing slowly and deeply can relax your body, clear your mind, and increase your ability to communicate effectively.

Deep Breathing Exercise

Begin by lying on your back, and relax body. Then inhale deeply and exhale fully. On the next inhalation place your hand on your stomach and note the region over your stomach expand as you inhale deeply. Keep taking deep breaths until you feel the region over your stomach expanding on the inhale and contracting on the exhale. Now, close your eyes. Imagine your body as a hollow vessel and every breath you take flows from your head down to the soles of your feet. Take your time and don't rush through this experience. This is time that you've set aside for yourself to simply enjoy the feeling of breathing deeply. The experience should feel comfortable and relaxing. Remain on the floor, simply breathing, for at least five minutes. When you feel that you've experienced deep breathing and allowed your body to relax into it sufficiently, row to the right side of your body and rest your head on your right arm, rest your left arm on the right side and stay in that resting position for a minute. Then using your left hand push yourself slowly and come into an upright sitting position. Stay in this position and continue to breathe deeply for at least a minute before getting to your feet. The deep breathing pattern in which you expand the region over your stomach on the inhale, and contract on exhale is the most natural, and efficient way for your body to breathe. With enough practice, this proper breathing technique will soon become second nature, and you'll find yourself speaking more comfortably and with greater confidence. In addition, performing deep breathing before the interview is very effective in keeping your mind clear and not wandering in thinking of things that'll increase your anxiety. Deep breathing will decrease anxiety and help you remain relaxed when you are waiting to begin your interview.

Exercise

Regular exercise is good for maintaining good health and keeping you from getting sick. So it is recommended that you engage in regular exercise at least three months before your interview. But do not suddenly start doing exercises within half a month of your interview as you will be placing stress on your body which will impair your performance on the interview. There may be a tendency to start exercising as you approach the interview to catch up on lost exercise time, or as something to do to improve your performance because you've exhausted all alternatives of preparation. But exercise needs to be done regularly for a period of time and cannot be crammed as many students have done prior to exams. You will probably have an irregular schedule for the few days surrounding your interview and may not be able to exercise at that time. Due to such practical limitations, it is probably better not to exercise for those days and if you manage to fit exercise in during those days, you should simply stretch or do yoga and treat that week as a rest or recovery week.

Two weeks before the interview

The last mock MMI, should be done within the last two weeks before the actual MMI and again should be video recorded. The last mock MMI should be done to most mimic the actual MMI conditions including the appearance of the room, the strict timing, and the process of entering and leaving the room per question.

Now when we review the performance of the last mock MMI, we'll be approaching the day of the real interview and it isn't the time to dwell minute details. The most valuable thing you can do for yourself now is to think of every good thing that happened during your mock interview and especially in terms of the progress you've made since your first mock interview. When you finish the last mock MMI and review the video recordings, only look and write down the strengths of your mock interview. For at least five minutes, write everything that comes into your head in response to this question: What was good about what you just did?

9. Special Section for Applicants Flying Out of Town to Prepare Prior to the Interview

This chapter is specially designed for applicants who are flying to another school for their interviews. If you're not flying to another place for your interviews, you can skip ahead to the next chapter. Many applicants will need to fly out of town to interview at different schools and there are many more preparations and considerations when leaving your home city. You want to minimize disruptions in order to have the most smooth interview and best conditions to help you perform at your peak on the day of your interview. That is the reason a special section has been dedicated to help you prepare and plan for your interview away from home. At the end of the section there is a list and description of essential things to bring or pack when flying for your interview to make each trip as easy and seamless as possible.

Preparation weeks before the interview

The moment you receive an interview offer, it is a good idea to book your hotels early because usually there are limited spaces and other students will be booking at the same time as well. It is not uncommon to have the hotels very vacant for the entire month but be full for only the few days that interviews are being held at the university. The same goes for booking interview time slots if the school offers that as an option. Interview time slots are booked at an amazing rate, where a quarter of the spots may be filled with minutes of releasing the interview notice. In general, booking plane tickets early will give you a good deal as the prices tend to increase or the flight times available become less appealing as the days tick closer to the actual interview date.

Preparation the day before the interview

The day before the interview should be planned to allow for time to relax and make preparations to feel ready and confident for the interview scheduled for the next day. There is usually enough time to get an idea of the city and school and to do some explorations on your own. You will uncover interesting things that won't be covered by the tour of the school and it will also help you ask questions about the school and city. At the end of the day, you will have two necessities that will make you feel comfortable and help you start the next day fresh –these would be a delicious dinner and a good night's rest and there will be some tips to help you make these two things happen as easily and smoothly as possible.

Getting to know the city of the medical school

If you arrive the day before the interview and you have time, it is an opportunity to explore and experience the city. An efficient way to experience the city or town is by taking public transportation from the airport to the hotel. It gives you an idea of the quality of the public transportation, a chance to experience the city as a local resident, a chance to see the city, a possibility to talk to the locals, learn about the city and medical school from the locals' perspective, and offers an adventure to learn a new public transportation system. If you plan to use the public transportation system, you should do some preparatory work while in your hometown by printing out all the relevant bus schedules and maps from the city's public transportation website, and having the routes planned out using Google Map and the city's public transportation website. To ensure you will get to your destination, you should have the hotel's contact information and map, the taxi phone numbers for the city printed and carries a cell phone in case you get lost on the way to the hotel. Some situations where it may not be advisable to use the public transportation system are if the town or city doesn't have a good connection from the airport to the hotel, if the city has a high crime rate, or if you fly into the city at a late time in that you won't have time other than to unpack, eat, shower, and sleep.

Dinner

Finding a place for dinner after you arrived in a new location is important. Most people will want to find a convenient location, low cost and usually something quick for their dinner. Finding a restaurant at different foreign cities for dinner can be very difficult, and often results in lots of walking, time, and drains your energy. In addition, it will often be fairly expensive, or have variable prices and types of food. Following with the theme of being in control of the situation despite changing environments and keeping your condition consistent, the best place to get food is at the airport. The airport invariably has a food court or fast food restaurants that provide low cost, quick, wide selection and convenient food. The moment you leave the airport, you are at risk of not knowing when you'll find another restaurant that you would want to eat and not knowing what kind of food or price you'll end up paying. You can usually find something healthy, filling, and low cost at the food court. A suggestion for convenient, healthy, and cost effective food court selections would be combination orders of rice or noodle with vegetables at most Chinese fast food restaurants. Orange juice or soft drinks are common and safe choice of drinks. These drinks are served in most places including on airplanes, have a good taste, provides rehydration, and is safe from complications of the gut. If there is a limited selection of restaurants, McDonald's is a familiar environment with known food selection and price. McDonald's is also a good place to fall back on because it often the last restaurant to close and a place to count on regardless of the time of day.

Sleep

Getting sufficient sleep is even more important when you are abroad and especially when there is a change in time zone. You want to aim for about ten hours of sleep prior to your interview. You may be jet lagged from flying in to your interview destination but the act of resting and lying on your bed in the dark for ten hours will ensure that you have attained the maximum amount of rest you can possibly achieve under your circumstances.

Setting a timer to wake up for the interview is important to wake up on time for the interview. Setting up multiple timers is a better idea. Sometimes one of the timers can fail or be set incorrectly and you would be at risk of being late for an interview. Setting up multiple timers is very easy to do in a hotel room. The most reliable and important timer is the watch you bring with you. You set the timer on your watch first. Then you set the timer on the clock in the hotel room to be one minute later than the timer on your watch. So when you wake up from the timer on your watch you can turn off the timer in the hotel room clock as well without being bombarded with buzzers.

Preparations for the day of the interview

Breakfast

If you are travelling outside your hometown for an interview, you have a couple of options to prepare breakfast. The first option is that you need to find a place to get breakfast the day before to ensure a seamless place to get breakfast. You don't want to be frantically searching for a place to have breakfast on the day of the interview. If you are at a hotel, they often provide free breakfast or there are breakfast restaurants nearby. This option is convenient but you are at the whim of the location and cannot control your breakfast intake. The second option is to bring a convenient and palatable breakfast so that you are in complete control of your breakfast. You control your nutritional value, time, and certainty of your breakfast. A suggestion for food to bring for breakfast that is portable, quick, and healthy is instant noodles. Instant noodles can be comfortable and convenient breakfast or can take place of any meal during an emergency. The hot water to make instant noodle can be obtained by boiling water in a percolator in the hotel room or hot water provided by the hotel. While the water is boiling you can begin dressing up for your interview. During breakfast, you can watch the news on the television to get the latest news in the place of the interview so that you have conversational information that you can use in the interview or you might learn new pieces of information that you can incorporate into your interview answers. The route from the hotel to the interview site should be mapped out prior to the trip on Google Map at home, and if you can walk to the site, you should walk the route the day before. If you plan to take the taxi, then you should book the taxi the night before the interview and give at least 30 minutes of buffer in case the taxi is late.

Importance of water and healthy snacks

Always carry a bottle of water on the trip to the interview site and on the flight to the destination. If you can't carry water on the plane, you can carry a disposable water bottle and fill the bottle with water when you clear customs and wait for your flight. It is important to stay hydrated throughout the day, so you will want to have a water bottle at your side on your way to the interview and during the interview. The medical schools almost always will provide the applicants with water but there have been cases when the water was provided late in the interview, the water was placed in an area difficult to access, or not enough water bottles. Water quality varies between cities and towns and it is usually advised to avoid drinking from the tap. Generally, the drinking fountains of airports are reliably clean but some people may not be used to the taste of water in some cities. Boiling water at the hotel with the percolator is an alternative to obtaining drinking water. For added comfort and personal choice you can bring your own tea bags and make tea by boiling water with the percolator. Drinking tea at night before you sleep or in the morning before the interview is a good way to calm yourself down, think about ideas that would be useful for the interview, and fill in those gaps of time when you are waiting in the hotel room.

On domestic flights, you can carry fruits on your carryon bags to use as healthy and cost effective snacks to keep your energy level up. In addition, granola bars or energy bars are compact sources of nutritional food that you can carry with ease when flying.

After the interview

You'll want to check in for your flight back and you can do that on a computer at the school or on a laptop and use the printers at the medical school or library. If you don't want to spend too much time at the school, you could go directly to the airport to check-in. A laptop is not necessary for interviews and may be a hassle as you will need to protect something valuable and have extra bulk and weight in your luggage. Computers are available at all universities in the student area or libraries, although you might not have 24 hour access to the internet, computer or printers.

A checklist of things to pack when traveling to an interview

When you have to travel outside your hometown for an interview, you generally want to pack light to make the travel as easy and stress free as possible. But you want to make sure you've pack everything you need to make you feel comfortable and prepared for your interview. A checklist of items of bare necessities to pack for short 1-3 day interview trips has been prepared at the end of this chapter.

Items to bring in jacket and traveling outfit

In keeping with the goal of traveling light, a strategy is to maximize the things that can be carried in your day clothes. Wearing a set of clothes during the day when you're not in the interview or sleeping eliminates a set of clothes to pack in your suitcase. The choice of day clothes depends on the season and should be comfortable. During the winter, suggestion for clothes to wear during the day includes a pair of warm sweat pants, a thin shirt, a sweater, running shoes and a waterproof winter jacket with lots of pockets to hold things close to you for accessibility and security. In the summer or spring months a similar ensemble can be used but the winter jacket would be replaced with waterproof jacket with many pockets and replace the sweater with lighter shirt. The jacket can hold many items that are valuable or you want ease of access. Some items that are suggested to be in the jacket include the passport, plane ticket, interview time information, directions to the hotel, MP3 player, eye glass case and wallet/change purse. The MP3 player is small and provides good entertainment for long waits at the airport. You can upload movies for anticipated long waits at the airport and listen to music, podcasts or audio books for shorter waiting periods. The headphones come in handy when watching movies on the airplane where most airlines don't provide headphones anymore. For people who wear glasses, the eye glass case is useful to protect your glasses when you want to nap without wearing your glasses. Other suggested items that can be easily carried in your jacket include pen, paper, napkins, and snacks/chewing gum. The pen and paper can be useful during unexpected events or simply to jot down gate information on connecting flights. The chewing gum is useful to reduce thirst and anxiety prior to the interview.

Items to carry in wallet

To minimize the risk of losing your wallet, you should place it in a pocket with a zipper or close off the pocket with a clip or safety pin. Try to minimize the valuable items and carry only the required number of identification. Some items to carry in the wallet include money, phone card, bus card, driver's license, credit card, and student ID card. The amount of money to bring should be calculated with about 30% more as a margin of safety. Remember to convert the money to the currency of the country, but also carry some money in the currency of the original country in case you need it. An example of an unexpected case would be the car breaking down en route to the airport and requiring money to take a taxi to the airport. The phone card is very useful and cost effective for situations in which you need to phone home or the university.

Items to bring in luggage bag

To avoid waiting and retrieving luggage at the carousel, you can limit your luggage to the maximum number of carryon luggage. Generally, the maximum carryon luggage allowed is two bags, such as a laptop or handbag (16cm x 33cm x 43cm), and one suitcase (23cm x 40cm x 55cm). The luggage of the stated dimensions will fit comfortably in the overhead bins of the airplane. Using only carryon luggage minimizes delays in finding and getting luggage after and between flights, and the possibility of luggage loss. The handbag can be used for two purposes, to carry daily required items on the plane and as a bag to carry to the interview site. The suitcase holds the interview outfit, toiletries and sleeping clothes. The handbag is versatile and is a convenient place to hold food and documents. For example, the handbag can hold a bowl of instant noodle for each day you're away, fruits if allowed by customs at the airport, notepad, pen, and interview documents that you may need to show at the interview. The suitcase can be used to hold your interview outfit, sleeping clothes, and toiletries. Other miscellaneous items that might useful are an all purpose container and bags. A thermally insulated multipurpose cup or bowl, such as a thermos, can be used to hold any hot or cold liquids. Plastic bags can come in handy to hold things, keep thing separate and to hold soiled clothing.

Other important items to bring

Other items to bring are a watch and cell phone. The cell phone duplicates the functions of the watch. Remember to charge the cell phone prior to leaving. The difference between the alarm clock function of the cell phone and watch is that the watch is less prone to running out of batteries and serves as the essential role of reliably providing the time and acting as an alarm clock.

The following page is a list and summary of all the items described and recommended for traveling abroad for medical school interviews. The list is divided by the container as the major headings for the suggested items to bring. Checkboxes are present beside each item to make it easy for you to keep track of items that you've packed.

List of Things to Bring

- [ ] Day Clothes
    - [ ] Sweater
    - [ ] Pants
    - [ ] Shirt
    - [ ] Casual shoes
- [ ] Handbag
    - [ ] Food, snacks
    - [ ] Fruits
    - [ ] Notepad
    - [ ] Pen
    - [ ] Interview documents
- [ ] Suitcase
    - [ ] Sandals
    - [ ] Tea bags
    - [ ] Clothes
        - [ ] Undergarment
        - [ ] Socks

- ☐ Interview Outfit
- ☐ Sleeping Clothes

- ☐ Toiletries
  - ☐ Toothbrush
  - ☐ Toothpaste
  - ☐ Deodorant
  - ☐ Hand Lotion
  - ☐ Chap Stick
  - ☐ Shaver (for men) or make-up (for women)
  - ☐ Cup
- ☐ Napkins
- ☐ Bags
- ☐ Multipurpose container

☐ Wallet

- ☐ Money
- ☐ Phone Card
- ☐ Bus Card
- ☐ Driver's License
- ☐ Credit Card
- ☐ Student Card

- ☐ (Winter) Jacket
    - ☐ Passport
    - ☐ Pen
    - ☐ Paper
    - ☐ Napkins
    - ☐ Snacks/Chewing Gum
    - ☐ Plane Ticket
    - ☐ Directions to hotel
    - ☐ Interview time information
    - ☐ Eye glass case
    - ☐ MP3 player
- ☐ Watch
- ☐ Cell phone

10. Preparation the day before the interview

Preparation before the interview is very important to ensure that you are at your peak condition. For the day prior to the interview, you should aim to sleep for ten hours. If you are not used to sleeping early in order to attain the ten hours of sleep, you should still at least be in bed and rest with your eyes closed to attempt to reach the ten hours of sleep and maximize your rest time prior to the interview.

At the end of the preparation and training, you've done everything you could do to prepare yourself for the MMI and you want to be relaxed so you can react to the spontaneous aspects of the MMI. So the few days prior to the MMI should be used to relax and reward yourself for all the hard work you've done to prepare for the MMI. You should be applauded for getting this far in your preparation and application process. Since there's nobody to applaud your completion of a long and arduous preparation, you have to treat yourself. It's an excellent way to relieve stress, refuel, and puts you in the best condition for the MMI. Here are some suggestions:

- Go out to a restaurant for a delicious meal
- Walk in a scenic area
- Get a massage
- Read a short story or a fiction you enjoy
- Watch a movie
- Take a nap
- Call or talk with a good friend or someone you miss
- Or any activity that you enjoy or find special

Taking time to take care of yourself is important, so try to do as many nurturing activities as you can, because you deserve it.

11. What to wear for the multiple mini interview?

In an interview you want to dress relatively formal to show you respect the interviewer and to give a positive impression. You also don't want to stand out in a negative manner compared to everyone else. A safe route would be to dress conservatively and not standout from everyone else. An alternative route would be to dress conservatively and modify the outfit by style or accessories to show something unique about you. This route can make you more memorable than everyone else or even give you a more positive impression than others but if done poorly it can give you a negative impression. In a traditional interview, making you more memorable has some advantages. But in an MMI, you are scored immediately after you finish answering your question and the interviewer doesn't think twice about you and will not be evaluating you after those minutes you were in the room, so being more memorable does not give you an advantage. If you can make you outfit standout to produce a better positive impression than others, you would have an advantage but at the risk of producing a negative impression and under the unknown subjective view of about a dozen different interviewers, it would be difficult to know definitely that your unique ensemble will produce a positive impression on every interviewer. Hence, barring superb fashion sense, it would be prudent to select a conservative outfit that doesn't standout too much from other applicants. For men, this generally leaves them with two options. The first option is classically conservative and involves a black suit, generally a white shirt, and a tie. The tie is generally blue but according to traditional colors, can be yellow or brown. The design of the tie should be simple, and striped designs are an innocuous choice. The drawback of a black suit is that it can be too serious and stifling. This leads to the next option of being formal and being comfortable at the same time. Men can wear a blazer and dress pants along with a shirt and tie. This ensemble is versatile in the combination of color and designs and is less stifling and serious than a black suit. A suggestion for the second option would be a navy blue blazer, gray pants, white shirt, blue striped tie, and black dress shoes with black dress socks. This is a classic and conservative ensemble that indicates respect for the interviewer while being formal without being pretentious or overbearing. The second option could also potentially make the interviewee standout from the other applicants while being respectful and formal at the same time.

Women have a wide selection of clothes they can choose from and they can be creative in their outfit and should aim to be respectful and formal. Women can get away with a wide ensemble as long as it is not too revealing and is relatively conservative. The two classic options many women often opt for are pant suits or blouse and skirt. In selecting a skirt, the skirt should not be shorter than knee height. Skirts are a prerogative for women and can properly distinguish themselves from the men and this means another tool or option that women can use at their discretion. It can make an outfit formal and comfortable at the same time and adds variety to an outfit much like the blazer option for men.

12. The day of the interview

On the day of the interview, you'll probably be most nervous when you're waiting in the room with other applicants and culminates to the moment you stand in front of the door with your back to the question. Chances are, despite your preparation, you're still a little nervous. That's a good thing. If you were totally relaxed, you'd be asleep and that would not make for a good interview. The interviewers will understand that the interview will be stressful and especially the multiple mini interview. Staff and students will be there to make the MMI as smooth and stress-free as possible and cradle you between questions to make sure no one will get lost and everyone knows what to do and expect. They won't hold nervousness against you, as you should to be a superhuman. It's a sign that you're taking the opportunity seriously. You can turn the nervousness to your advantage by channeling the extra energy into the interview. The higher heart rate pumps more blood to your brain so you'll be more alert and react faster than usual.

Here are a few tips to help you perform at your best on the day of your interview:

- Allow yourself plenty of time to get ready before leaving for the interview. You need to allocate enough time to comfortably wake up, make breakfast, dress up, and commute to the interview location. You should have about 30 minutes of buffer time and arrive at the interview about 30 minutes early.
- Take your time getting dressed. Make certain you look your best so that you'll feel your best.
- Remember, if you've made it to the interview, you are a selected few and the medical schools want to meet you.
- Finally, know that you are now in the best possible physical and mental shape to succeed in this interview. The MMI is more fun than a standard panel or job interview. Enjoy yourself.

13. After the interview

Congratulations! You've completed the multiple mini interviews, and that's no easy task. During the interview, everyone was in the moment, consumed with the immediate concerns of completing the interview. Afterward the interview is the time for reflection. Keep a journal of your answers, progress, and questions asked after each interview to monitor your progress and to stimulate you to think and prepare for subsequent interviews. Think about what went well, and what didn't. Write in your journal for at least five minutes without stopping. What would you do the same in your next interview? What would you do differently? Did you present yourself in the best possible light? Did you communicate well? How did you do? The best time to do this is while you are waiting on your way home, or at home after the interview. If you flew away from home for the interview, a good time to reflect would be while you're waiting for your flight home and during your flight. You can type away with your laptop or enjoy the intimacy of writing your reflections in a notebook or journal.

14. CONCLUSION

You've now been introduced to the style of multiple mini interview questions and have an idea of the experience of an MMI and preparations that'll give you confidence in completing your own MMI. There is a full length practice MMI exam near the end to give you a chance to tackle the MMI and become familiar with MMI style of questions. Medical School Multiple Mini Interview: Full Length Practice Interviews is another publication with several sets of full length MMI exams designed to mimic the real MMI and this will give you more practice and develop a better sense of the experience along with the stress of a series of questions given in rapid succession. Practicing with many MMI questions will help loosen your brain and prime your brain to react and respond to a variety of MMI questions. I wish you luck in your multiple mini interviews and your admission for your medical professional career.

FULL LENGTH MULTIPLE MINI INTERVIEW PRACTICE

Full Length Multiple Mini Interview Practice

Below is a sample multiple mini interview that mimics the type of questions, duration and number of questions you would expect in an MMI. You should simulate the testing and room conditions described in this book.

Instructions:

There are eight questions. You have two minutes to read and think about the question and eight minutes to answer the question. Flip to the next page to view the prompting questions. Prompting questions are available on the next page and should be consulted when necessary. To best simulate the MMI, the interviewer will read the prompting questions when you've finished answering before the time limit or if you request for the prompting questions. Interviewer score sheets are provided at the end of the book. Cut out the interviewer score sheet and give it to the interviewer to evaluate the interview.

Flip the page to begin.

Q1.

You are a sales associate at Future Shop and you are teaching two newly recruited sales associates to be knowledgeable about the products and to provide excellent customer service. Both of the sales associates reluctantly listen to you and are not motivated to learn about the products and make no effort to help the customers. You are expected to train them in three days and your performance in training these rookies may be rewarded with a promotion. One of the new sales associates is the daughter of the manager and the other new sales associate is her friend.

How would you handle this situation?

Q1 Prompting Questions

A. What would be the first thing you would do in a situation like this?
B. What is the relevance of the new employee being the manager's daughter?
C. Is there a difference between how you would handle this situation in the short and long term?
D. Do you have any responsibility for the poor performance of the new employees?

Q2.

Your uncle and auntie are in their late 40's and have been trying to have a baby for the last twenty years. They've tried everything possible but were unable to conceive. Recently, a physician has developed a technique that will allow them to have five babies. They know you have a medical background and want to talk to you first.

How do you respond to your uncle?

Q2 Prompting Questions

A. What are the risks of operation?
B. What people are involved in this situation?
C. How does your uncle feel?
D. How do the other people in this situation feel?
E. What factors do they need to consider?
F. What are the consequences of their decision?

Q3.

You are on a Caribbean cruise ship that sunk and you escaped on a life raft. You are floating at sea on a life raft with enough room for three people. You have a box of food that takes up one passenger seat and you take up one seat so you have room for one other person. Your life raft floats towards two people wearing life vests floating in the water. One of the people in the water is a 12 year old child and the other is an elderly person. There is only enough space on the boat to take one passenger.

What would you do in this situation?

Q3 Prompting Questions

A. What are your options?
B. What other information do you want to know?
C. What emotions do you think each of the people involved is experiencing?
D. What would you do if you can only save one person?

Q4.

You are volunteering as one of the towel personnel for the diving competition at the Olympics. You've been diligently passing out towels to Olympians and enjoying the events. You have a towel in hand as usual and in the waiting area where the Olympic divers for Canada are waiting for their turn. You notice one of the Olympians started to cry. The Olympian is in the waiting room.

What would you do in this situation?

Q4 Prompting Questions

A. What would be the first thing you would do in a situation like this?
B. What are the consequences of him doing well or poorly?
C. How does the athlete feel?
D. What would you expect your emotions to be immediately after making your decision?
E. How could this situation be avoided?

Q5.

You mother is diagnosed with breast cancer and is deciding between surgically removing the entire breast and surgically removing a portion of the breast followed by chemotherapy. Removing a portion of the breast allows for most of the breast to be intact but chemotherapy has side effects that include loss of appetite and hair loss. The removal of the entire breast is more invasive but may not require chemotherapy. Both methods have similar chances of recovery and life expectancy.

What would you suggest for your mother?

Q5 Prompting Questions

A. Who is involved in making this decision?
B. What are some possible consequences of making the decision?
C. How do you feel about the decision?
D. How would your mother feel about the decision?
E. What factors do you need to consider?
F. How would you respond if your mother is hesitant about the operation?

Q6.

Your roommate has been dating a girl for five years. His girlfriend has been obliging and has been doing most of the household chores and they've been living together for two years before he moved in with you for university. He had to move away from home for university and they've been maintaining a long distance relationship by communicating online and see each other for a few days or week at a time when he visits his parents. Suddenly, your roommate's girlfriend tells your roommate that she wants to break up and your roommate is devastated.

How would you respond to your roommate?

Q6 Prompting Questions

A. How does your roommate feel?
B. What are some of the reasons for the sudden break up?
C. What are some options that your roommate can pursue?
D. What are the consequences of carrying out these options?
E. What can you do to help him?

Q7.

If, as part of the admissions process, we were to interview your best friend, what would they say about you?

Q7 Prompting Questions

A. What would they say would be best characteristic that you possess?
B. What would they say would be your weakness?
C. If you could change one thing about yourself, what would it be?

Q8.

A major drug company released a new method to administer insulin by inhalation. Insulin is normally administered by injection. Administering insulin by inhalation will remove the need to inject insulin. The experts have been debating over the benefits and drawbacks to the new inhalational administration of insulin. You are a family physician with a patient with diabetes and is in your office enquiring about receiving insulin by inhalation. The patient has a friend who is using the new method of administration and wants to try it.

How do you respond to the patient?

Q8 Prompting Questions

A. What are the considerations before you can prescribe this medication?
B. What are the benefits and drawbacks of delivering insulin by injection?
C. What are the benefits and risk of delivering insulin by inhalation?
D. How does your patient feel?
E. What options do you have in responding to the situation?
F. What actions would you take?
G. How do you ensure the patient understands the risks?
H. If the patient understands the risks and strongly wants the inhalational medication, will you prescribe the pain medication?

Comments for MMI Questions

Each MMI question is made to be open and can encompass a wide range of answers that are unique to each person. There are a few areas to note in providing your answers that will lead you to fulfill the points that interviewer is expecting and evaluating. These notes are provided for each of the questions in the practice interviews. At the end of the interview when you are reviewing your answers in your head and watching your answers on video, read the notes to ensure that you are on the right track and have incorporated the notes to provide the optimal answer.

Q1. This question is an attempt to create a creative scenario that is not entirely foreign to the general applicant pool. This question tests your ability to prioritize and to create a plan under a stressful and time constrained environment. Factors that need to be balanced includes the teaching of work ethic, teaching customer service, maintaining the company's reputation, methods to rectify the problem of lack of motivation, interpersonal skills in dealing with subordinates, communication skills that involve tact between you and your supervisor and subordinates, and justice and fairness in dealing with the consequences of improper action on the job.

Q2. This question is an opportunity to demonstrate your empathic, diplomatic, persuasion and communication skills. Some people may be emotionally involved in this question and maintaining composure and calmly analyzing and answering the question while at the same time being empathic, compassionate and understanding may be a challenge to some people. Age, culture, personality, commitment/drive for 20 years, other family members, ability to care for the children at such an old age, the children may not be able to experience a normal childhood because the father and mother will be too old to play sports and take them out, the cost to society of orphanage if the parents decide to abandon, the cost to the health care system if the techniques fail or have side effects. The technique is illegal in Canada but legal in the states. Your uncle and auntie are considering having the procedure done in the US. Another consideration is the cost for any side effects will be paid for by Canada even though it is not allowed in Canada and not by the US which was the country that performed the procedure.

Q3. Question 3 attempts to test your critical thinking skills and attention in reading the question. You can demonstrate your interpersonal skills, compassion, empathy, diplomacy and tact in your answer as you respond to the situation and make your decision. An ethical consideration may be lurking in your decision that you may need to deal with if you or the interviewer brings it up. Added to the mix is the consideration of the different parties involved, their interests and the consequences that can severely impact the survival and group dynamics. There are a number of options and some of them are innovative and requires some lateral thinking. One of the possible solutions is to recognize that you can have a person floating while hanging on the raft and take turns being in the water. Some people may consider throwing the food overboard in order to save another person but this opens up the question of the group's ability to survive and how long they can survive without food. Some questions that might ask for more information could be to consider if the box of food can float or if the people can use the life vest to float the food or to tie the food to the raft using some of their clothes. These solutions do not need to exclude or choose a person to save. The applicant should note that they are in warm waters because they are in the Caribbean and both of the capsized passengers have life vest and are not in immediate danger of drowning. Since you are floating in a boat while they are floating in a life vest in warm water, they are not necessarily in greater danger than you. There are probably more immediate dangers such as the passengers starving or having an illness that would pose a more immediate risk that should be dealt with first. There are a number of factors that need to be considered before one can make a decision of which person to save, including age, health of the two people, survival experience, the personal opinions of the two people themselves, and etc. Variations in these factors can significantly affect the survival of the people involved.

Q4. In this question, a creative scenario is created and this may surprise inexperienced applicants. The thought process and logic of the answer is primarily being evaluated by the interviewer. Your values and priorities that guide your decisions will be noted. The Olympian is very nervous and under a lot of stress and pressure because the next dive will determine whether or not Canada will get a medal or not. He has been receiving a lot of pressure from his friends, family, team mates, and coaches to do well and is often told in the media to be expected to bring Canada a medal from the Olympics. The second issue is that the pressure is getting to him and a child hood fear of heights is causing him to tremble and he is afraid to go out and dive. A possible response could be to go and chat with the Olympian and demonstrate empathy and active listening. Offer comfort and encouragement. He has been diving for many years and has been able to suppress his childhood fear of heights and the emotion and pressure at the moment is giving him doubts. By providing compassion, empathy, supporting him through encouragement and listening to him you will calm him down and he will emotionally de-escalate and be able to perform as he has flawlessly been diving for many years in preparation for the Olympics.

Q5. Question 5 involves being aware of the different parties involved, being empathic, being immersed in a personal situation, and weighing personal values, beliefs, and interests of different parties. There is some medical context but the scientific information isn't the emphasis. This situation is delicate in requiring the ability to be logical in the decision making process to analyze and be compassionate while being enveloped in an emotional and personal situation. This is a complicated question that should also implicate other family members. Other family members can also aid in consoling the patient and can help in facilitating a decision with mother if she is uncertain or hesitant. The psychological impact of the decision and alteration to the patient's self image and identity are significant factors to consider. The level of suffering she would need to endure for the consequences of either decision needs to be weighed. Chemotherapy has a different type of consequence that includes dealing with losing weight, not being to enjoy food and taste, the ongoing treatment sessions, and the gain of an intact breast is balanced with hair loss and emaciation. The decision is further complicated by the emotions of fear, shock, uncertainty, and confusion by the many people involved. The ability to be empathic intertwined with the ability to think logically in this tender scenario.

Q6. Your ability to provide compassion, empathy, and communication skills are tested. The incident is traumatic to the roommate and he is devastated and overwhelmed with emotions that may include confusion for the sudden break up, pain or heartache from the break up, sadness when he realizes the loss of someone he cares, self pity if he begins to blame himself for his girlfriend leaving him, anger that his girlfriend left him, or despair if he believes that he won't find another girl who would be as perfect his ex-girlfriend. There may be a number of reasons for the sudden break up and this could be due to accumulated stress of a long distance relationship that resulted in the last straw that broke the camel's back. There may be factors of under appreciation of the efforts or sacrifices made by the girlfriend. You can brainstorm reasons and possible solutions and options he can pursue and this will engage his mind in searching for solutions and analysis. He may be emotionally overwhelmed and not ready to think and analyze the situation, in which case, more time will be needed for him to calm down and you can listen and empathize with him. Some possible options include encouraging him to communicate with his girlfriend to better understand the situation and act on more complete information. If he feels that stress of a long distance relationship was placing a lot of strain on him too and he may even be considering the thought of breaking up. If he wants to continue with relationship he may be able to plan for the future with his girlfriend and salvage the relationship. On the other hand, if he chooses to break up it may be a tough decision for him to make but it may be better in the long term if there were deep rooted problems in their relationship. Sudden changes in his relationship causes undue stress and is a risk factor for depression that may spiral in mental illness. He needs someone to be there, support him, and to talk and listen to him. You would empathize with him and actively listen. You may suggest he look into counseling services offered by the university. You might try to engage him in social events to take his mind off of things and to provide momentum to get over the break up.

Q7. A certain level of self awareness is expected with the MMI and a lot of the MMI questions attempt to delve into you personally in an indirect manner. This question is considered a more direct approach in an attempt to understand the applicant and is not usually encountered in the MMI. However, this question stimulates you to think about characteristics of yourself that you may be able to consciously make shine in other MMI scenarios.

Q8. This is an involved question where ethical principles are also included in this question in addition to critical thinking, analysis and decision making. An approach in analyzing this problem is useful in answering this question. The ability to analyze and weigh the risk and benefits is important. The advantages of administering insulin by injection are that many patients are already trained with this route of administration, we already have specialized needles that painlessly and effective administer insulin, and that it is a method that has been used for a long time and we're familiar with the long term effects of this route of administration of insulin. The drawback is that injection is a relatively invasive technique and requires training. The inhalational route of administration has the benefit of being able to be administered non-invasively, requires minimal training, is quicker and more portable. Some considerations are that this new method of administration could have long term consequences that we don't know, especially since we're administering a protein into the delicate regions of the alveoli, the level of variability that an inhalation would consistently administer the correct dose, and the cost the new device for administration. The level of experience and comfort with injecting insulin, the reasons why the patient wants the new route of injection, and knowledge of the risk and benefits of inhalational insulin, need to be considered before you can make a decision. The level of maturity, exposure to injection and inhalational routes of administration, the patient's ability to relay the information conveyed and appreciate the consequences of the each route of injection are factors that should be taken in account in determining the patient's level of understanding. After balancing the risks and benefits, the values, beliefs, and lifestyle of the patient, and the patient's own decision and autonomy needs to be respected as well in making the final decision.

Interviewer Scoring Sheets

Instructions:

Cut out the interviewer scoring sheets and give it to the interviewer to evaluate and grade your performance. The interviewer will provide a grade from a scale of 1 to 10 ranging from poor to excellent for each category and an overall score. Space is provided under each category to note areas of strengths, challenges, and improvements.

MMI Score Sheet

Date: ___________________

Communication Skills:

Question #:	1	2	3	4	5	6	7	8
Score (__/10)								

Strength of Arguments:

Question #:	1	2	3	4	5	6	7	8
Score (__/10)								

Suitability for Health Sciences:

Question #:	1	2	3	4	5	6	7	8
Score (__/10)								

Overall:

Question #:	1	2	3	4	5	6	7	8
Score (__/10)								

REFERENCES

Eva KW, Reiter HI, Rosenfeld J, Norman GR, An admissions OSCE: the multiple mini-interview, Medical Education 2004a; 38:314-326.

Eva KW, Reiter HI, Rosenfeld J, & Norman GR, The ability of the multiple mini-interview to predict preclerkship performance in medical school, Academic Medicine 2004b; 79:S40-S42.

Eva KW, Reiter HI, Rosenfeld J, Norman GR, The relationship between interviewer characteristics and ratings assigned during a Multiple Mini-Interview, Academic Medicine 2004c; 79:602-608.

Eva KW, Reiter HI, Where judgment fails: pitfalls in the selection process for medical personnel, Adv Health Sci Educ Theory Pract 2004d; 9: 161 -1 74

Harasym PH, Woloschuk W, Mandin H, Brundin, Mather R, Reliability and validity of interviewers' judgments of medical school candidates, Acad Med 1996 71:40s-42s.

Reiter HI & Eva KW, Reflecting the relative values of community, faculty, and students in the admissions tools of medical school, Teach Learn Med 2005; 17(1):4-8.

GET MORE PRACTICE WITH

3 FULL LENGTH MULTIPLE MINI INTERVIEWS

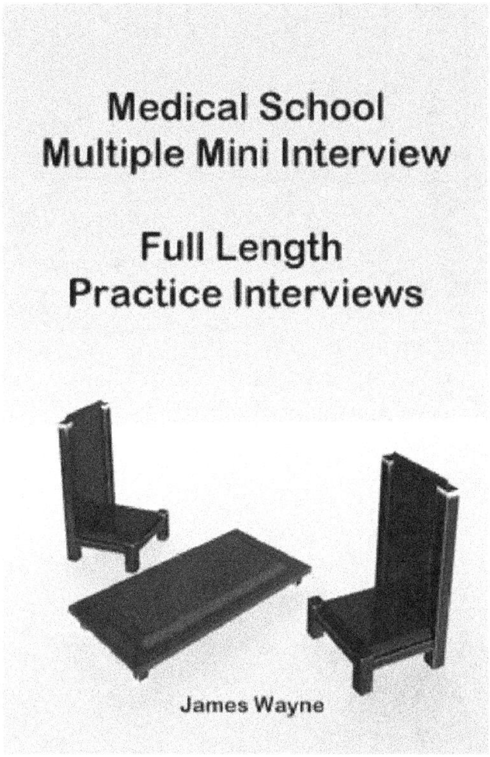

The question types are designed to stimulate the thought processes in the MMI and the appearance of the questions are made to mimic what you will see in the actual MMI. The practice MMI's include prompting questions that are asked by MMI interviewers. Discussions are available for each of the questions to check if your answers are hitting the areas the interviewers are evaluating and to stimulate you to provide fuller answers.

To order visit http://www.medicalschoolmmi.com

NOTES

NOTES